12 Practical Steps to a New You Forever

12 Practical Steps to a New You Forever

"From Shame and Sadness to Sheer Bliss"

Authors Francisco M. Torres, MD, Board Certified & Ashleigh Gass, MS, CSCS, CCN, CNS

Editor Abby Campbell, BSc, SFN, SSN, CPT

12 Practical Steps to a New You Forever: From Shame and Sadness to Sheer Bliss

ISBN-13: 978-0692385760
1. Health   2. Nutrition

Library of Congress Control Number: 2015933433

Version 1:1
First Printing February 2015
(paperback edition, 5" x 8")

Authors: Francisco M. Torres, MD, Board Certified & Ashleigh Gass, MS, CSCS, CCN, CNS

Editor: Abby Campbell, BSc, SFN, SSN, CPT

For more information including quantity discounts, please visit www.ForeverYoung.MD.

Dedication

This book is dedicated to all those who are working on managing weight for a healthy lifestyle. Your perseverance encourages us. When times get tough, remember that you can and will win.

Thrive to be forever young!

About Dr. Torres

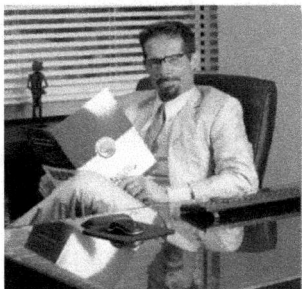

Dr. Torres specializes in the diagnosis and treatment of patients with spine-related pain syndromes and osteoarthritis of multiple joints. He has authored and co-authored several articles published in various medical journals and has also participated in several clinical research studies. His experience is vast:

- University of Puerto Rico (Cum Laude, BS Biology)
- University of Puerto Rico School of Medicine (MD)
- Veterans Administration Hospital, San Juan (Residency)
- Louisiana State University (Musculoskeletal Fellowship)
- American Academy of Physical Medicine and Rehab. (Member)
- American Association of Electro-Diagnostic Medicine (Fellow)
- International Spinal Injection Society (Member)
- American Board of Physical Medicine and Rehabilitation (Cert.)
- American Board of Electro-Diagnostic Medicine (Certified)

- American Board of Pain Management (Certified)
- International Spinal Injection Society (Certificate in Discography)
- Florida Academy of Pain Management (Past Vice President)
- Osteoporosis Program of Florida Spine (Current Director)

Dr.Torres is also the President and Medical Director of ForeverYoung.MD. As a trained age-management physician, he works with patients on preventing age-related disease in order to optimize health and longevity.

About Ashleigh

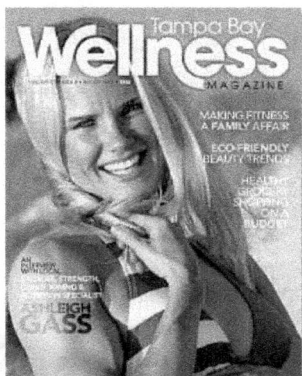

Ashleigh has been in the exercise physiology field for over 10 years. Her first degree was in Kinesiology and Exercise Physiology, from The University of Victoria, in her native town of Victoria, British Columbia, Canada. She completed her first graduate degree at The National Coaching Institute, and then her Master's degree in Clinical Nutrition from The University of Bridgeport, Connecticut. Her education is extensive and ongoing:

- Medical Exercise Specialist (MES)
- Certified Strength and Conditioning Specialist (CSCS)
- Certified Sports Nutritionist via The International Society of Sports Nutrition (CISSN)
- Certified Cross-Fit Trainer (CCFT)
- Certified Clinical Nutritionist (CCN)
- Certified Nutrition Specialist (CNS)

Ashleigh offers a host of services which include nutritional education, strength and conditioning training, and injury prevention training.

Table of Contents

*"Don't reinvent the wheel;
turn it into the landing gear
of a spaceship."*

~ Dr. Torres

Introduction

Perhaps some readers will approach this eBook as just another one of the thousands of eBooks that are out there covering topics of health, weight loss, and physical transformation. Perhaps you have arrived at this page still holding on to some doubt or fear, however much, suspecting somewhere deep inside that you're on the brink of yet another let down.

The power to change your life for the better is in your hands right now. Life transformation isn't the stuff of fairy tales and misplaced hope. Instead, life transformation is real and it's for you, no matter what your own story is or who you may be.

The logical possibility of physique change is clear. Most people understand that the human body has the capacity both to store excess fat and burn that fat off. Nutrients can be measured. Metabolic rate can be calculated.

The fogginess is purely mental. Beaten down by the oppressiveness of obesity and all that comes with it, some people have stopped believing they can change. Jaded by past failures, they hide their fear in cynical skepticism.

Whatever your current state is, or your past, don't let it define you. You are your potential.

Don't worry about whether or not you believe you can change. Logic doesn't require your belief. Expect progress instead, as you follow this program.

From Shame and Sadness to Sheer Bliss

I (Dr. Torres) wasn't always the muscular medical expert that I am today. Instead, I spent most of my life reeling from the effects of childhood obesity. For almost four decades, I felt like a victim. Like most people who are overweight, the related shame and physical limitations cast an oppressive pall over my life, preventing me from pursuing many of my ambitions.

In fact, I vividly recall the pain and embarrassment I felt. I shied away from my favorite sports. I lacked the confidence to be social. I panicked at the thought of taking off my shirt for pool parties and at the beach. That isn't easy for someone growing up in Puerto Rico. My physical appearance took a devastating mental toll.

Extreme physical consequences followed. One day, I found myself hospitalized and facing cardiac catheterization. Afterwards, I began to realize just how much pain and suffering being overweight was causing. I suffered, but so did those patients of mine whose bodies were in similar condition.

I became determined to act. No longer could I sit idly by and watch obesity consume any more of my life. I decided to pour my focus into making a change for the better and helping others do the same. My research combined with my medical knowledge allowed me to design the wellness lifestyle which set me free. I am decidedly no longer a victim of obesity!

Today, I am fit and healthy. It has truly been a transformation. Not only did I lose the weight and gain 6-pack abs, but my emotional and social health has improved even more significantly. I have a better relationship with my family, my patients, and myself.

Many of the tools I used to exchange lifelong shame and sickness for sustainable vitality and bliss, I want to share with you in this eBook. If I can do it, then anyone can, including you!

From Debilitation to Deliverance

This isn't an eBook just about weight loss. Although the regimen featured is highly effective in correcting obesity, this eBook is mainly about achieving optimal health. Even those whose goal isn't to lose weight can benefit from practicing the 12 steps.

For example, consider the experience of Ashleigh Gass, a new partner in the business of providing ultimate wellness. She's a high-level athlete, expert nutritionist, and highly competitive Certified Strength and Conditioning Specialist (CSCS). On the surface, Ashleigh seems to be the last person who would need to undergo a transformation.

But severe back pain has plagued her for almost half of her life. In fact, it was recently that Ashleigh's sudden neurological deficits caused her to require immediate back surgery. Imagine one of your lumbar discs re-herniating, splitting downwards into the spinal cord, shutting off sensory and motor nerve supply to the lower leg and foot.

While some may have required extensive recovery time after undergoing such a surgery, it took only days for her to recover to the point that she was able to return to gym training. In fact, leading up to neurosurgery, she never stopped. Just a few months later, Ashleigh not only competed in a physique show, but she placed second overall and in her respective divisions. The difference between her recovery time and that of the average patient was due to several factors:

1) Excellent neurosurgeon (Dr. Chris Mickler).

2) Re-training her back, as well as her knowledge of spinal training to include Foundational Gymnastics Training through Coach Chris Sommers. *(You'll read about the importance of joint mobility in this eBook.)*

3) A lifetime of health practices and nutritional strategies outlined in this eBook. *(Literally, Ashleigh's body can recover from anything thanks to her robust health.)*

Out of the Dark and Into the Light

No more quick fixes! The results that quick fixes produce, if any, vanish just as fast as they come. They often leave the user worse off than they were before. There are dire consequences to poor lifestyle and eating habits, and avoiding those consequences means changing those habits.

So many shy away from any advice that tells them to make a permanent change for the better because they're afraid of the commitment, somehow assuming they'll be forced to swear off what they enjoy and be sentenced to a life without pleasure. Ironically, it's this fear that keeps them firmly in obesity's grasps, which indeed is life on the unpleasant side.

A lifestyle of health is a rich lifestyle. What shall you accomplish when you're physically fit, healthy, and far more confident? You become limitless.

Moreover, the pleasure of eating doesn't get taken away. You just learn to eat smarter so that your body works together with you in achieving your goals, instead of working against you. As you follow the fitness routine you'll discover that you have more energy, strength, and are able to do more of the things you enjoy, and that equates to a fuller, richer life.

The following 12 steps are designed for smooth integration into even the most hectic lifestyle, leaving everyone who reads this eBook without an excuse. As well, you'll find that making the transformation you desire isn't a matter of willpower as much as it is about simply having and using the right information.

The time to set free that grand version of you that's been hiding in the shadows of obesity and/or poor health is right now. Let the true you step forth into the light not just so that everyone else can see it, but so that you yourself can bask in its glory.

You've come this far. Don't let procrastination stand between you and your brand new self. Start with step 1 right now.

PART I: Setting Yourself Up for Success

✓ *Attaining Your Goals*
✓ *Keeping a Food Diary*

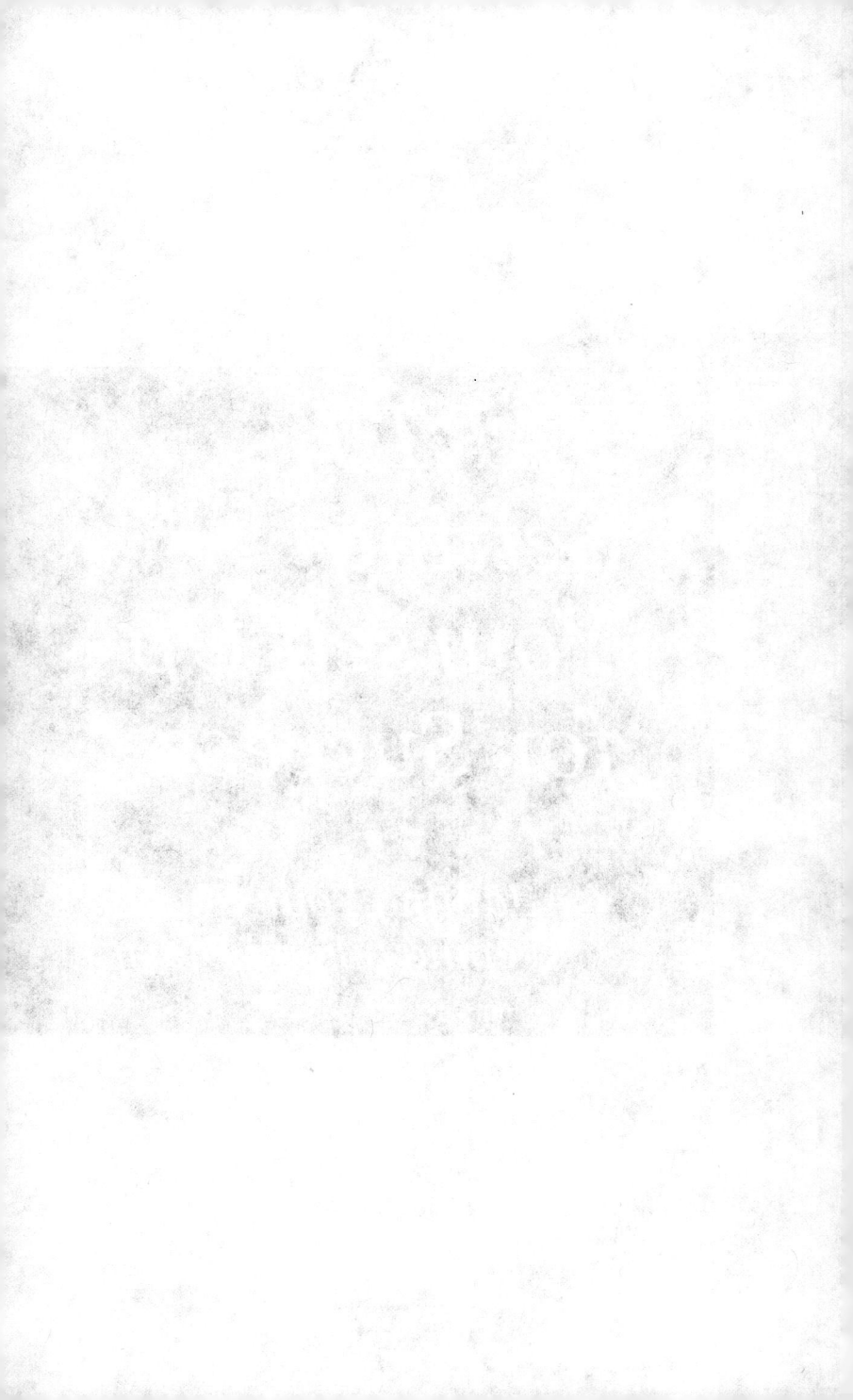

STEP 1: Attaining Your Goals

Of all the different factors that must come together in order for you to reach success in the achievement of your goals:

Motivation!

Your motivation is king. Although many people who want to lose weight consider themselves sufficiently motivated, what makes all the difference is being able to stay motivated enough to remain on track day in and day out. Your success depends on it.

If you want to stay motivated throughout all the little changes and hurdles life may throw your way each day, you have to take the time to meditate and reflect on your goals each and every day. This keeps your goal, and the reasons for wanting to achieve your goal, at the forefront of your mind.

In fact, focusing too much on progress might be a big mistake. Some people become discouraged when they look at the progress they've made each day and find that they're not moving forward as fast as they think they should.

Focus on your goals every day and you won't go wrong. Even in the most discouraging times, you'll be able to stay motivated.

Weight Loss: The Mental Game

It's true that many people fail to lose weight simply because they've employed the wrong strategies. Things like eating the wrong carbohydrates at the wrong times, for example, can block weight loss results.

But the most determined and motivated person will not yield to failure. They will continue on until their goal is achieved. They will make continuous progress, finding solutions instead of quitting when they think they've gone wrong.

Knowing what to do is a lot different from actually doing it. It's not until the knowledge is applied that the benefits can be received.

Therefore, weight loss is very much a game of mental strength. However, it isn't necessarily the one who's naturally strong-willed that makes it, as much as it is the person who will look upon their goals each day and reflect. Therefore, we encourage you to think deeply and carefully about your own goals.

Goal Reflection: Your New Good Habit

With a food log, you can keep track of your workouts, your carbs, and even how much water you drink. Be sure to keep track of your goals and motivation as well.

Write down your goals. Moreover, make note of your reasons for having these goals. If you happen to find some quotes that inspire you, put them there right along with your goals and reasons.

Review this information frequently. Reflect on your goals each morning, each night, and even in the afternoon if you can.

Not only does the frequent review and reflection of your goals help you stay motivated. The more you review and reflect on them, the more ingrained they become in your mind.

When goals aren't reviewed often, you run the risk of forgetting what the true focus of the day is. The motivation that was once so great tends to deflate. We don't want you falling off your plan for days, weeks, months, and even years before attempting to get back on track.

After a while, you may find that when you're challenged to make the right decision for your health, or when an obstacle which may throw you off track is placed in front of you, you'll instantly take the path which progresses you to the achievement of your goals.

Action Step

Take time daily for quiet reflections of your goals. Refine them, make adjustments, and stay the course. Create a sleep routine (see Step 11). This quiet time, at night, may be your best starting point to calm down and reflect on your goals for the next day.

STEP 2: Keeping a Food Diary

Keep a food and beverage diary for a few days!

The things you eat and drink have an impact on your life. What you consume affects more than just your health and body weight. It also affects your mood, energy level, and more. Depending on what your current nutritional habits are, even small gradual changes can result in large changes that have a positive impact on all aspects of your life.

Without much consideration of what current habits are, some people are anxious to change their eating and drinking habits without transition. This can cause failure, and no one wants to fail in achieving goals. Without a smooth transition, one can revert back to old habits. Even worse eating and drinking habits can occur thanks to subconscious rebellion. Rather than shocking your system into sudden change, we recommend a gradual transition in order to maintain good habits for a lifetime.

Some people have trouble changing their dietary habits simply because they don't see what's wrong with the habits they have now. You might be surprised what the diary will reveal about you and your choices. It's also a good way to track your progress when changing so that you can take note of and congratulate yourself for small achievements.

Catch Yourself in Your Habits

Keep a written food and beverage log for one week. You may surprise yourself and say, *"Wow, I didn't realize I was doing THAT!"* Write it all down. After all, it's just for one week!

Clients and patients often tell us how healthy they eat. We discovered this has varieties of meaning – anything from Raisin Bran for breakfast, donuts for snacks, store-bought wraps for lunch, cans of soda or energy drinks for afternoon cravings, and the first good meal of the day at dinner. As you may guess, erratic patterns and lots of processed foods lead to some pretty sick folks.

Once people actually see their patterns, they come back to us rather shocked. At this point, we are more effective as practitioners to begin adding things to our clients' deficient diets. You too can keep track of your foods and beverages which will help you determine where you need change. This diary can also help your physician, nutritionist, or trainer should you choose to work with one.

How to Start and Maintain a Diary

We've had people track their food intake with notebooks, phone apps, or personal computers. We're fine with either, granted it's as accurate as possible.

Thanks to modern technology, there are many options you can use to track what you eat. We recommend the phone app *Lose It!* where you can log your foods meal by meal, set goals, and check how you're doing for the day. The app even provides you with calorie information of many built-in foods which saves you time. However, you can customize your foods as well. Best of all, the app is free!

You may also obtain *Lose It!* through your desktop or laptop. Setting up an account is free, though a premium membership may be obtained for only $39.99 per year. Just go to www.loseit.com. *(Please note that we have no affiliation with the app or program. We just find it to be a great approach for tracking.)*

Even though there are great digital tools for tracking your food and beverages, the old-fashioned notebook journal is sometimes best. If you choose this method, you may want to use a small journal for discretion. Set your notebook up in the following columns or rows:

- Morning Weight *(after emptying bladder & before first meal)*
- Meal Number
- Time Eaten
- Food Consumed

Write everything you eat and drink in this diary. Also, track how you feel for the day. Were you lethargic? Were you moody? Did you have any allergies, hives, or rashes? Have you lost weight? Write it all down. These things are important as you'll be able to look back and see what works and doesn't work.

Action Step

Create a food and beverage journal. In can be a notebook, phone app, or personal computer program. Track your weight, meals, and anything else that will help you manage your weight and become healthier.

PART II: Healthy Eating for Success

✓ Water
✓ Protein & Carbs
✓ Starchy Carbs
✓ Low-Glycemic Carbs
✓ Fat Versus Sugar
✓ Portion Size

STEP 3:
Water Versus Calories

Get rid of useless calories and drink more water!

You might assume that if you're already logging what you eat and how many calories you consume, it's totally redundant to consider fluids. However, there's more to it than you might think. We've encountered people who drink diet soda, energy drinks, and coffee all day in an attempt to *ramp themselves up*, or sadly, to replace meals. Both are major mistakes in the long run, having significant negative impacts on body fat and the endocrine system.

What's So Bad About Caloric Liquids?

First thing in the morning after training, a caloric protein shake is favorable on the body as it provides it with nutrients. Your body loves it as it is being restored after exercise depletion. However, sodas and sweetened teas are loaded with refined sugars that don't provide your body with any benefits. They are *useless* calories.

Your body keeps track of the calories you consume, but it doesn't treat all calories in the same way. Rather than taking in 150 *empty calories*, your body would better appreciate you for the extra 150 calories in solid and wholesome food. Your brain just won't register *fullness* with the empty calories consumed in liquid form, and you most likely would end up eating more in the end. It would be a great mistake to assume juice, milk, or energy drinks as being as healthy as natural and whole foods. Ultimately, any calorie you drink just ends up being excess calories.

You may choose to drink alcoholic beverages when you go to social events. Though we believe that this can negatively affect health and weight loss if consumed too often, we will keep it real here. Most people do enjoy a social drink or two to help them relax. If you do, choose less sugary forms and avoid adding juice or tonic water as they just add calories to the already calorie-filled drinks.

Plain purified water is best for your body. If that sounds boring to you, try flavoring it with some small slices of your favorite fruits. Fruit is very nutritious, and it's very refreshing as well. You'd be surprised!

Aren't Milk and Fruit Juice Healthy?

Milk and fruit juices are touted as being good for the body. We often hear about their nutritional benefits. It's thought that calcium from milk is a way to fight osteoporosis. Some even think that vitamins from fruit juice ward off disease.

Though you may obtain some vitamins and minerals from milk and fruit juice, numerous studies show that natural and whole food is more beneficial. Most people drink milk for its calcium and vitamin D content. But, did you know that both spinach and salmon provide even higher amounts of calcium? You can also obtain more than enough vitamin D by just being in the sunshine for 20 minutes per day.

Instead of fruit juice, the actual fruit can be eaten instead. This not only allows you to benefit from the vitamins and other nutrients fruit contains; it also lets you benefit from the fruit's fiber, which can help you stay feeling full longer.

There is one argument floating around for drinking juice as it's claimed that juicing fruits and vegetables release more nutrients to help the body better absorb them. However, that's exactly what chewing does – helps release nutrients into the body. Be sure to always chew your food well.

Why Is Water Best?

The body doesn't always differentiate between thirst for water and hunger. Because of this, it's very easy to overeat. However, you'll experience less of this mixed message if you consume enough water in a day.

Giving your body enough water helps to ensure it works at optimal level. Water is essential to flushing out excess fat and waste. Best of all, water is filling. The list of health benefits water provides is great:

- carries nutrients and oxygen to cells
- protects organs
- regulates body temperature
- lubricates joints
- moistens mucous membranes
- helps kidneys and liver flush waste

Best of all, water helps reduce your cravings for sugar-filled foods and beverages.

How Much Water is Enough?

Did you know that the average adult loses about 10 cups of water a day? That's just one of the reasons that the old *8-glass* rule simply doesn't work. There are other factors that can also significantly increase the amount of water you need to drink daily.

One important factor needed to calculate the amount of water you should drink is your weight. Take your weight and multiply it by 0.67, which is 67 percent. After you've multiplied your weight, the resulting product is the number of ounces of water you should normally drink.

Body Weight

x 0.67

===============

Ounces of Water

After calculating your water needs by your body weight, you will need to add more for your activity level. For every 30 minutes of strenuous activity in your day, add 12 more ounces of water to your daily water intake.

Try to replenish the water your body naturally loses each day. An easy way of keeping track of how much water you drink each day is to simply record it in your food and beverage diary.

Action Step

Calculate your water needs. Record it in your food and beverage diary. Mark off what you drink each day. Make sure you get what you're supposed to in order to ward off the sugary cravings for empty calorie drinks and food.

STEP 4:
Protein & Carbs

Get enough protein and control your carbohydrates!

Many people just assume they're getting enough protein and would be surprised to find out that such isn't really the case. While many dishes contain meat which are high in protein, other meals may not be high in protein. We see many deficiencies in those who live off of processed and pre-packaged foods.

While recommended daily caloric intake is based on the age and sex of a person, proper protein amount is calculated by body weight and activity level. There could be a big gap between the amount of protein you get and how much you should really have.

If you're a sedentary adult, you can optimize your weight loss by making 30 percent of your diet protein. If you exercise on a regular basis, your protein needs may increase to 1 to 1.5 grams per pound of lean body mass weight, depending how strenuous your workouts are.

Protein-rich foods include beef, chicken, turkey, fish, eggs, cottage cheese, and Greek yogurt. Whey, hemp, pea, and amino acid powders are also quick protein sources and great after workouts. Other foods which contain some protein but also have higher carbohydrate or fat content are lentils, beans, nuts, and cheese.

How Protein Helps Weight Loss

Protein helps to support lean muscle. When losing weight, this means you'll be able to maintain more muscle rather than lose muscle along with fat.

Protein is also made up of amino acids, and amino acids are highly effective at revitalizing a sluggish metabolism. Muscle burns fat, and amino acids boost metabolism, making the consumption of enough protein fundamental to healthy and effective weight loss.

What About High Protein & Low or No-Carbohydrate Diets?

Since protein is so great for weight loss, and many are warned to avoid consuming too many carbohydrates, shouldn't an only-protein diet be the most logical and effective choice? Many doctors, nutritionists, and trainers recommend a high protein, low carbohydrate diet. In fact, some recommend a protein-only diet. However, that's actually not the most logical and effective choice.

We'd like to point out that there are many benefits to carbohydrates in the diet. The brain and central nervous system prefer glucose for fuel, and muscles use it for recovery. While the body can produce glucose from amino acids (via a process called gluconeogenesis), the estimated amount is about 50 grams, which may or may not be enough depending on your level of activity.

As a general strategy, we recommend the bulk of your carbohydrates come from greens, salads, peppers, zucchini, carrots, beets, and other colorful vegetables. However, we also recommend adding starchy carbohydrates immediately following strength training to help your body recover faster (*more on this in the next step*). Starchy carbs include yams, sweet potatoes, squash, and gluten-free grains such as brown rice or quinoa. Quinoa is one of the grains naturally higher in amino acids.

Carbohydrates are food for your muscles and essential for proper brain function. Without them, your memory will suffer, and so will you. In fact, the functioning of the entire body begins to decline when it doesn't get the carbohydrates it needs, resulting in negative side effects such as muscle cramps, weakness, diarrhea, bad breath, and more. Finally, thyroid function will suffer causing a slower metabolism and can even cause metabolic failure.

Even though we don't recommend the low- or no-carbohydrates diets, that doesn't mean you shouldn't control the amount and quality of incoming carbohydrates.

Action Step

Include protein in every meal and snack throughout the day. An easy method is to measure quality protein by the palm of your hand. Athletes may need more. Also, include lots of cruciferous and colorful vegetables. Limit starchy carbs for after workouts which is roughly a 50 gram serving.

STEP 5: When to Eat Starchy Carbohydrates

Save your starchy, high glycemic carbohydrates for the anabolic window!

As mentioned in the previous step, carbohydrates are naturally an important part of the human diet. Going completely without them can result in a number of health issues, so the real issue with carbohydrates should be timing.

The improper consumption of starchy carbohydrates is one of the main causes of numerous cases of obesity. Insulin is the culprit behind carb woes, as it is the hormone that acts to store carbohydrate energy in fat cells. Whenever the average person consumes carbohydrate-containing foods (especially those carbohydrates that are starchy and high glycemic), their body reacts by secreting insulin into the bloodstream.

However, storing the energy from carbs as fat is not the only action insulin can take. Instead, there is a time when insulin stores that energy in muscle cells. That time is called the anabolic window.

What is the Anabolic Window?

The anabolic window is the best time to consume any carbohydrates that are starchy and high glycemic. This timeframe occurs directly after intense physical activity (such as a high intensity interval training (HIIT) workout) and lasts for about 45 minutes to two hours.

In fact, if you want to lose weight and gain or maintain muscle, you should consider it the only time to consume such carbs. This is the best time as insulin stores carbohydrate energy as glycogen instead of fat.

Glycogen is a form of glucose that is stored in muscle, which causes muscles to be plump and feel solid. More importantly, the body uses glycogen as a form of energy more readily than it uses fat. Intense workouts deplete your muscle's glycogen stores, and it seeks to refill them afterward.

Because glycogen stores of energy help to prevent muscle loss, it is important to assist the body in replenishing that glycogen. As mentioned previously, the time immediately after your workout is your window of opportunity.

Carbohydrates are the food for muscles. Without enough of it, muscles turn to amino acids contained within themselves as a source of energy. This leads to muscle loss, as well as fatigue.

Why Are Starchy Carbs Best During the Window?

Foods higher in starchy carbohydrates during the anabolic window essentially help the body shuttle nutrients straight to muscles. Foods such as sweet potatoes, potatoes, rice, and quinoa fit into this meal. By taking advantage of the window, glucose tolerance is increased. This aids recovery. Just be careful to not go overboard in consuming too many carbs during this time, and stay within the guidelines of your caloric target.

Insulin reaction to consumed high glycemic carbohydrates can work against a person whose goal is weight loss. This is especially true if those carbohydrates are consumed outside the anabolic window. However, those same carbohydrates can assist the person in goal achievement when they are consumed within the window.

That is why we stress the window of opportunity for starchy carbs being after workouts or other high activity. The anabolic window is the only exception wherein eating high glycemic carbs is beneficial to those whose goal is weight loss. During any other time, be sure to stick to low glycemic carbohydrate sources, mainly vegetables and fruit.

Action Step

Include starchy carbs after a strenuous workout only. This includes foods such as sweet potatoes, potatoes, rice, and quinoa.

STEP 6:
When to Eat Low Glycemic Carbs

Stick to low glycemic carbohydrates on non-training days!

The anabolic window becomes accessible to you on the days that you train, and that's the best time to reap the benefits of eating high glycemic carbohydrates without experiencing the fattening downsides. But what about the days you don't train?

By now, you realize that the actions of insulin can be both beneficial to you and also harmful. Yet, not all carbohydrate-laden foods cause the same insulin response. The difference is in the sugars these foods either contain or can be derived from.

How Are Low Glycemic Foods Measured?

First, let's take a look at a few different measuring tools used to determine the sugar load in foods:

- Glycemic Index (GI) - measures how quickly and significantly a certain food raises blood sugar

- Glycemic Load (GL) - based on the GI multiplied by the serving size of food

- Insulin Index (II) – predicts the insulin response to a meal by measuring the insulin response to a food directly

Both GI and GL have their limitations while the II is useful in measuring.

If you were to eat a meal composed of white potatoes, salmon, and kale, the GI would register quite low. This is due to the high protein and fat content in the salmon as it stimulates a greater insulin response. If the potato were measured alone, the GI would be quite high.

Low Glycemic Carbs Versus Starchy Carbs?

For fat loss, you should focus on carbs with lower GI and II for the majority of your meals. Practically speaking, this means eat salads and vegetables throughout the day. If you're training hard, we encourage you to add higher GI foods like a white potato or ripe banana to the first meal post-training.

Though you may recognize cookies, cake, and ice cream as being high glycemic or sugary foods that can lead to fat gain, you may be surprised at the healthier options. Many natural foods are considered high glycemic: watermelon, ripe bananas, pumpkin, dates, and russet potatoes. However, these high glycemic foods are better on insulin response due to fiber and other nutrients that cookies, cake, and ice cream don't have. Nonetheless, save these healthier options for your post-training meal, when your body can take advantage of higher insulin levels.

Such surprises are the things that prevent many from losing weight, despite their best efforts. If your goal is to lean out and lose fat, you don't need starchy carbohydrates on non-training days. However, the body still needs some carbs every day in order to have sufficient energy. Cruciferous and colorful vegetables would suffice.

On some days, the demands for energy are much higher than other days. Therefore, feel free to eat high glycemic carbohydrates during the anabolic window, but make sure you stick strictly to low glycemic index carbohydrates on the days you don't work out. Stick to carbohydrates that have a low glycemic index, such as the wondrous amounts of vegetables and fruits such as grapefruit, plums, peaches, berries.

Action Step

On non-workout or rest days, include low glycemic carbs to your diet such as vegetables and fruits like grapefruit, plums, peaches, and berries. Stay away from starches.

STEP 7:
Fat Versus Sugar

Isn't Dietary Fat Bad?

It's a common misconception that dietary fats are responsible for weight gain. In fact, it's only been relatively recently that researchers have realized some high-fat foods are actually beneficial to health and weight loss.

Natural dietary fats are important to health, and they are categorized as:

- saturated
- monounsaturated
- polyunsaturated

Though all these fats are equally important to your body, they are not all created equal.

Even saturated fats? Yes, even saturated fats are important to your health. In the past, it was touted that saturated fats were bad in that they increased cholesterol which contributes to heart disease. However, recent scientific studies indicate otherwise. In fact, saturated fats (specifically palmitic, myristic, stearic, and lauric) raise HDL (good fats), lower cholesterol, and may even help with weight loss. It's not that saturated fats are bad, but eating them in excess is what causes issues (*refer back to calorie overload being the problem*). Now that you know the truth, you no longer have to be afraid of eating beef.

With that being said, monounsaturated and polyunsaturated fats have long being known to contribute to health. Specifically, a type of polyunsaturated fat known as Omega-3 has been reigned king of the fats for its many health benefits. Not only does Omega-3 ward off heart disease, lower cholesterol and inflammation, and promote healthy cells, brain, and nervous system. It even helps with weight loss.

Monounsaturated and polyunsaturated fats (including Omega-3) foods include olive oil, olives, avocados, flaxseed oil, flax seed, chia seeds, walnuts, and cold-water fish. Salmon, tuna, mackerel, herring, sardines, and anchovies are great sources of cold-water fish.

You can now throw out the old assumption that dietary fat is bad and causes weight gain. When it comes to obesity, the real problem with fat (*as well as starchy carbs*) is its high calorie content. Generally speaking, you can eat fat safely as long as you stay within your calorie limit. Overall, *natural* dietary fats are an important energy source.

How Much Sugar is Too Much?

Like dietary fat, overconsuming sugar will cause health issues. Even though it is possible to stay within your calorie limit when eating high glycemic foods, you can still gain weight.

As WebMD reports, research is continuing to mount on the case against sugar consumption by those seeking weight loss. A study published in *The BMJ Journal* (2013) showed subjects who stayed within their calorie limit gained weight while consuming sugar. However, those in the study who did not consume sugar actually lost weight.

It may be obvious that candy, cakes, and cookies contain refined sugar. But, did you know that even eating high glycemic carbohydrates also convert to sugar in the body? This includes breads and pastas. It may even include those natural starchy carbs like sweet potatoes and rice. Eating these high glycemic carbs can have the same effect as eating those sugar-laden foods commonly known to be unhealthy.

Action Step

Don't be afraid to include natural dietary fats to your diet, especially Omega-3. Stay away from refined sugar.

STEP 8: True Portion Size

Resist the temptation to supersize!

Eating at fast-food restaurants can be a problem for those who eat at fast food restaurants. It can also be a problem for anyone prone to *better buys* or anyone who has the mentality that *more is better*. We've been taught to save our money and to obtain as much as we can for as little cash as possible with most things in life. However, economics is different when it comes to food. More is not always better.

The sentiment that *more is a better value* could get you into big trouble when it comes to calories. Not only can super-sizing meals result in calorie overload, but it doesn't necessarily help you save money or get more of anything that's good for you.

With the rising cost of healthcare, you need to take care of your body. What seems to be saving pennies now can actually break your bank by thousands when the medical and prescription bills begin piling up due to poor eating. It's time to get in the habit of being happier with less food so that you can have more of what you really do want, and that's a healthier and functioning body as you grow in age.

The Virtue of Learning Portion Size

Healthy foods such as lean protein and low glycemic carbohydrates must be consumed only in proper portions. Controlling portion size is a habit you can learn, but staying within your daily recommended caloric intake can prove difficult.

Though many foods come labeled with nutrition value and how many servings are within the package, it can still be difficult to figure what that serving or portion size is when divvying up. For example, you can prepare a meal for your family using a bulk package of chicken breast.

The label may tell you that 8 servings at 4 ounces each are contained within the package. But, can you actually tell what the proper portion size is when you dish the chicken out of the pan onto your plates?

Even more difficult can be divvying portion size when there are several ingredients. Ever wonder about portion size when you go to buffet style dinner? It may not be feasible for you to swear off going out to eat, but it is reasonable for you to learn how to control your portion size.

Making sure to log the food in your diary before you eat the meal may help. It forces you to take a hard look at the food you've put on your plate. However, developing an insightful eye for portion size can keep you from disrupting your diet at times when you can't make diary entries.

What Does a Portion Size Really Look Like?

The meals at restaurants aren't always the single portions nutritional guidelines dictate. In fact, most of these meals are found to be two or even three times the recommended serving size.

Many people have become accustomed to over-serving, and being over-served, that it would be easy to consider a true single portion as too small. As a result, regularly overeating may not even be realized.

For protein servings, the size of the palm of your hand is a good measurement. To determine serving sizes of carbohydrates, ask yourself if you've trained for the day. If you answered *yes*, then have a serving of starchy carbs such as a medium-sized sweet potato or yam. If you didn't train, choose from many cruciferous and colorful veggies. Serving size loses importance when it comes to most vegetables and salads. Just choose your favorite whether it be spinach, kale, broccoli, tomatoes, or peppers. There are hundreds of veggies to choose from.

Keeping Tabs on Your Plate

A simple way to keep from overdoing portions is to use a smaller plate. More importantly, you must avoid the temptation to help yourself to more servings.

Earlier, we discussed super-sized meals when eating out. If and when you must dine out, get into the habit of ordering the small size or dividing your plate into two meals. Share one of the meals with whomever you're having dinner with, or save it for another time.

Wouldn't life be much easier if you didn't have to worry about what you were going to eat each day? One of the best ways to make sure you're controlling meal portions is to plan ahead. Stock your refrigerator, freezer, and pantry with healthy foods. Prepare many meals at the same time, so you don't have to worry about what you're going to eat with time crunches. Preparation is one of the keys to successfully living healthy.

Action Step

Be conscious of what you eat. Make portion control a habit. Use your palm to gauge protein portions. Eat starchy carbs only after workouts. Eat as many cruciferous and colorful veggies as you want. When eating out, order the small size or divide your meal.

PART III: Healthy Exercise & Rest for Success

✓ *Lower Body Strength*
✓ *High Intensity Cardio*
✓ *Flexibility*
✓ *Rest & Healing*

STEP 9:
Lower Body
Strength

Focus on building a strong lower body!

For those who are overweight and seeking to slim down, the abdominal muscles are often the main focus of training. In fact, training this muscle group is even a primary focus for those who are not even obese, as the gut is a common problem area. While it's true that a greatly protruding belly can be unattractive and a sign of poor health, placing too much focus on training the abs and not enough focus on training other areas of the lower body is a strategy that can backfire.

It may even be great to have lean, ripped arms, shoulders, and pectoral muscles. However, the importance of upper body strength pales in comparison to having a lower body that's lean and strong.

The lower body is a major source of power and strength for the entire body, and many problems result from it not being well trained. Focusing on strengthening the lower body includes working on the muscles of the lower back, hamstrings, gluteus (your butt), and calves. Not just the abs!

Too Much Abdominal Training is a Problem

There are many benefits to having strong and lean abdominal muscles. Fit abs provides better posture and a lower risk for cardiovascular disease. However, the result for those who focus too much on training the abs can be low back pain along with other ailments. This includes those who love to perform abdominal exercises every day.

Focusing entirely on the abdominal muscles can leave the lower back exposed to weakness. Excessive tension is created in the lower back if this area isn't trained along with the abs. The abdominal muscles then pull on the lower back, which creates imbalances between the two groups.

Moreover, the presence of belly fat isn't a reliable indicator of abdominal muscle strength. Those who have abdominal fat and judge their bodies based on appearance alone may assume that abdominal strengthening is the remedy they need, but such a conclusion may be far from true.

Though abdominal exercises may require a lot of work, many produce minimal results to reducing belly fat. Without a proper nutrition plan and cardio regimen, the fat will still cover the muscles underneath.

The Benefits of Building a Lean Lower Body

Your lower body is the foundation of your body and a major source of power. It includes some of the largest and most used muscles. Even better, strengthening these muscles can help your body naturally burn more calories per day.

Having a strong lower body is an important key to improved athletic performance. It is also essential to performing many everyday activities, such as walking up the stairs. If you're seeking weight loss, strengthening this area will help you perform certain routine activities that you may not have been able to do before. This is a clear signal of improved health.

Moreover, strengthening and building your lower body muscles will also boost your metabolism which will help you achieve your weight loss goals.

Strategies for Lower Body Training

When training, many people perform body part exercises by isolating single muscles. An example of this would be bicep curls where the biceps are trained with little strength building of any other muscles.

A better way to train is functionally where multiple muscles and joints are worked together. An example for a functional exercise is the squat. Squats specifically target the gluteus, quads, and hamstrings in the lower body. However, this exercise also trains the rest of the body, including the back and abdominals.

The deadlift is another excellent move for strengthening the lower body. This exercise move uses several muscles in the back, as well as the gluteus, hamstrings, quads, and calves. Bridging exercises performed from a ball or flat bench are excellent progression moves to prepare the body to deadlift.

Please be sure to learn these movements from a certified strength and conditioning specialist or trainer. Formation is very important for body improvement as well as keeping yourself from getting hurt.

Action Step

Learn how to train your lower body. Work with an experienced coach to learn how to train using exercises such as squats, deadlifts, and lunges (as well as all variations of these exercises). Instead of focusing on direct abdominal exercises, integrate core training in with your lower body training weekly.

STEP 10:
High Intensity Training

Perform high intensity interval training!

One of the main reasons many find it difficult to achieve their weight loss and health goals is an inability to stick to an exercise regimen. Yet regular exercise is essential to producing the desired results.

Maybe you are one who simply finds workout programs boring. Or, are you discouraged because the exercises are too hard? Sometimes, it's just difficult to find the time due to so many demands in life.

Staying with a program for months can be tedious. Plus, it can be very discouraging when visible results aren't produced in what seems to be a reasonable amount of time.

Whatever your issue may be with exercise, don't feel bad. There have been plenty of athletes and coaches who also fall short at some time or another. Unfortunately, life sometimes just gets in the way.

However, developing an effective exercise strategy can help. High intensity interval training (HIIT) is a strategy that may help with not only time but also with results. Besides, it can be fun!

What Exactly is HIIT?

The basic principal of HIIT is alternating between high and low intensity and speed. When compared to other cardiovascular exercises, such as *steady state* cardio rhythms, interval training results in greater fat burn. However, HIIT allows users to exercise for shorter periods of time and still receive better results than they would otherwise. Research shows that HIIT can help you effectively burn fat even when you're resting. While regular steady state cardio burns fat during the exercise itself, HIIT helps your body continues burning for 16 to 48 hours *after* the exercise.

According to an article published in the *Australian Family Physician Journal* in 2012, HIIT greatly enhances weight loss benefits. This exercise strategy even proves superior for producing a number of other health benefits such as lowering the risk for cardiovascular disease and stroke. It also lowers blood pressure, improves cardiovascular health, and improves metabolism and endurance. With HIIT, we've found our clients to be leaner and metabolically healthier in all areas including inflammatory markers and hormone profiles.

How to Do HIIT?

Whether you prefer working out at your local gym or at home, you must find the right HIIT workout that's suitable for your fitness level and lifestyle. It is a fairly simple process.

For those who prefer to exercise in the privacy of their own home, numerous HIIT workout videos can be found. DVDs can be purchased online or locally. However, you may also find free workouts on YouTube as well. By following a video, you just have to follow along without paying too much attention to the clock. For beginners, this can be a relief.

However, if you prefer working out at the gym, or are simply uncomfortable following exercise videos, there are many ways you do HIIT, and you can even Google free exercise charts online. HIIT can be done just about anywhere, as long as the basic principles are adhered to. That includes the intervals, speed, and intensity.

To do HIIT properly, you will begin with a short warmup at low to medium intensity. Then you will alternate a short period of high intensity exercise followed by a short period of low intensity exercise. This alternation will continue for several cycles. After you've completed these cycles, you will cool down at a low intensity speed for a few minutes. The entire session can range from 10 to 30 minutes depending on your fitness level.

Perceived Exertion Scale

A way of measuring intensity level for physical activity is by using a *Perceived Exertion Scale*. Perceived exertion is how hard you feel like your body is working. It is based on the sensations you may feel while exercising. This includes increased heart rate, breathing rate, sweating, and muscle fatigue. Although the scale is a subjective measure, the rating may provide you with a fairly good estimate of the actual heart rate while exercising. On the next page, you may find a scale to use while performing HIIT.

Rating	Description
0	Nothing
0.5	Very, Very Light
1	Very Light
2	Light
3	Moderate
4	Somewhat Hard
5	Heavy
6	Heavy
7	Very Heavy
8	Very Heavy
9	Very Heavy
10	**Very, Very Heavy**

Example 1 – Using an Elliptical

Remember to use the *Perceived Exertion Scale* above when performing HIIT. Level 1 will be very low intensity while 10 is very high intensity. On the next page, you will find an example for a beginner with 11 minutes of HIIT and four rounds.

Intensity / Speed	Minutes
Warmup (Speed 1-4)	3 minutes
High Intensity (Speed 7-10)	30 seconds
Low Intensity (Speed 2-4)	1 minute
High Intensity (Speed 7-10)	30 seconds
Low Intensity (Speed 2-4)	1 minute
High Intensity (Speed 7-10)	30 seconds
Low Intensity (Speed 2-4)	1 minute
High Intensity (Speed 7-10)	30 seconds
Low Intensity (Speed 2-4)	1 minute
Cool Down (Speed 1-3)	2 minutes
Total	**11 minutes**

Example 2 – Using a Recumbent Bike

Again, remember to use the *Perceived Exertion Scale* on page 65 when performing HIIT. Level 1 will be very low intensity while 10 is very high intensity. On the next page, is an example for a moderate to advanced trainee with 23 minutes of HIIT and five rounds.

Intensity / Speed	Minutes
Warmup (Speed 1-4)	3 minutes
High Intensity (Speed 7-10)	2 minutes
Low Intensity (Speed 2-4)	1 minute
High Intensity (Speed 7-10)	2 minutes
Low Intensity (Speed 2-4)	1 minute
High Intensity (Speed 7-10)	2 minutes
Low Intensity (Speed 2-4)	1 minute
High Intensity (Speed 7-10)	2 minutes
Low Intensity (Speed 2-4)	1 minutes
High Intensity (Speed 7-10)	2 minutes
Low Intensity (Speed 2-4)	1 minutes
Cool Down (Speed 1-3)	5 minutes
Total	**23 minutes**

The most frequently used methods of HIIT include cardio equipment such as the elliptical and recumbent bikes presented above, as well as treadmills and stair climbers. However, HIIT can be done without a machine such as with running the track or bleachers. Jump squats, burpees, and mountain climbers can also be done by using your own body weight – no machines required. It can even be completed with resistance training by alternating between weightlifting and cardio (where cardio is the high intensity portion).

Though each HIIT session finishes with a 2 to 5 minute cool down, you want to make sure that you continue cooling down with flexibility or mobility training. This will help your muscles from cramping and your blood from pooling. (*More on this will be discussed later.*)

How Much HIIT?

Because of the sudden bursts of fast-paced and intense movements, as well as the many options available, HIIT workouts are less boring. However, HIIT does require you to put forth your maximum effort.

If you are a beginner, you may want to start with very short periods in alternating times as well as total time. Example 1 (above) is a great starting routine, though it may be much if you have been sedentary for a very long time. Therefore, you may want to start with short high intensity and longer low intensity cycles. Also, you may want to begin with two sessions per week and spread out with three days in between. Your endurance will improve with time, as well as your physique.

The body adapts fairly quick with exercise. Therefore, it's wise to change your routine every four to six weeks if you're using the same HIIT approach each time.

Exercise Tip

Try to exercise outdoors. The sun exposure will help anchor your circadian rhythms which will help you sleep better. Twenty to 30 minutes will provide you with sufficient amounts of Vitamin D which will also help with weight loss efforts.

STEP 11: Flexibility Training

Improve the mobility of your joints!

Good joint mobility is an important factor of both fitness and overall health. Improving your joint mobility can make it easier for you to:

- perform a number of activities
- increase your fitness level
- aid prevention of disease
- lose weight

Ever tried putting your shirt on when you can't lift arms overhead? How about being able to bend over to put your socks on? Rather valuable life skills, we think!

A loss of flexibility is one of the earliest signs of aging. Many find that with age, they can no longer do the agile moves they could once perform in their youth. Being less flexible has also contributed to weight gain in some, as the immobilization of joints reduces circulation. Experiencing discomfort, when performing certain movements, has inspired them to settle for a more sedentary lifestyle. This lifestyle is not good for the joints as they are meant to help you move. Many repeatedly walk and sit, but rarely do they rotate or extend. Mobility training is one of the keys to reverse aging, and it may require a good coach to help you implement a valuable flexibility plan.

Flexibility and Exercise Recovery

Increasing the range of motion of your joints helps reduce your workout recovery time while boosting your athletic ability. These benefits can greatly assist in accelerating you towards the achievement of your weight loss goals.

A slow recovery time from workout sessions is one factor that has caused many to fail in achieving their goals. Let's face it! It's tough working out at the next session when you are still hurting from the last. Because of that pain, have you ever felt you couldn't continue? All because of slow recovery, many have actually quit their exercise routines after discouragement from non-recovery.

It can take several days to recover your tight muscles and joints from a strenuous workout. Adding flexibility training helps as it will help with recovery time. Shorter times of recovery will also help you get back to your training quicker which also allows you to burn more calories and fat.

Ways to Increase Your Flexibility

Joint mobility can be increased in a variety of way. Stretching, and mobilizing connective tissue, is the underlying focus of each physical activity. This increases the range of motion of your joints.

Certain exercises provide great flexibility approach. The practice of yoga is an effective approach to enhancing your flexibility. Yoga will also help with strength gains, weight loss, and stress relief. Foam rolling can be done without a trainer. It is a self-help technique to assist you with soft tissue and muscle recovery.

When exercising, warmups and cool downs are also very important. Warmups *before* exercising will help lubricate your joints and activate your muscles for strenuous exercise. Stretching *after* a workout improves joint mobility and assists in the prevention of injuries.

Action Step

Begin mobility and/or flexibility training weekly. This may entail going to a yoga class, taking a flexibility class at your local gym, or dedicating two nights a week to foam rolling.

STEP 12:
Healing & Rest

Develop a healthy sleep routine!

The stress and demands of modern day life have left millions of people sleep deprived. Day in and day out, we are on the go without any recovery or downtime. People generally don't pay attention to their sleep until it's seriously affected.

Regularly getting a good night's sleep is essential to overall good health, well-being, and weight loss. Sleep researchers have proven that chronic sleep deprivation influences everything from decision making to reaction time, the ability to focus on one task at a time, and food choices.

Sleep Deprivation & Weight Loss

Appetite

When you are sleep deprived, you are more prone and susceptible to food cravings. This can quickly drive up your calorie count for the day. Seeking out supplemental energy is the case for many with fatigue. Consuming energy drinks, extra carbohydrates, or caffeinated and sugary sodas will halt weight loss progress.

Sometimes, this isn't completely a conscious or controllable choice. One of the negative impacts of sleep deprivation is an imbalance of hormones. Higher ghrelin (hunger hormone) and lower leptin (satiety hormone) may cause overeating. Your body enters into a state of *metabolic grogginess* wherein it no longer uses insulin efficiently. This also leads to weight gain.

Training

If you are able to exercise when sleep deprived, your performance may not be up to par. Sleep deprivation leaves you with low energy which may make it difficult to get through your training. Worse yet, you may be too tired to workout at all.

Cloudy judgment from lowered cognitive functioning can put you at greater risk for injury. Cortisol (stress hormone) may also interfere with tissue repair. This makes it difficult for your body to recover from the workouts as it should.

Technology's Effect on Sleep

With the busy world we live in, it may be difficult to get the rest you need. After all, we live in a world of technology. Phones are beeping every few minutes, and the internet is available 24 hours a day. A study by the Lighting Research Center (2012) declares that two hours of "self-luminous electronic displays can suppress melatonin [sleep hormone] by about 23%" while also disturbing the circadian rhythms. Additionally, your brain's feeding center goes into overtime. This causes hunger which leads to overeating.

Televisions, computers, and mobile phones all emit light. By interacting with them before bedtime, your brain is constantly reading the light. One of the best things you can do for yourself is TURN OFF these electronic devices. By allowing your body and mind to transition from daytime mode into sleep mode, your health and weight loss efforts won't be in vain.

Appropriate Amount of Sleep

The need for sleep is different for each person. While the National Sleep Foundation recommends adults get seven to nine hours of sleep each night, you may have to gauge what is best for you.

Though the amount of sleep is important for health and weight loss, the quality is just as important. Avoid the negative effects of a chaotic schedule where you're going to sleep at a different time each night. The *American Journal of Health Promotion* (2014) found that this variation, even by 90 minutes, can affect body fat. For someone whose goal is weight loss, that information should serve as a great motivator for developing and sticking to a healthy sleep routine.

Building Your Sleep Routine

If you're having difficulty sleeping, now is a good time to build a quality sleep routine. Following is a plan you may want to utilize:

1) Turn off all electronic devices at least two hours before you plan to go to bed.

2) Drink an herbal tea called *Sleepytime* made by Celestial Seasonings. It contains a blend of chamomile, spearmint, and lemongrass which

provides calmness and prepares for sleep.

3) Sleep until you wake up naturally in the morning. If you don't wake up before your alarm goes off, go to bed a little earlier the next night. Once you are awaking naturally before your alarm, make this your normal bed time. Record the hours you've slept for a few nights. This will tell you how much sleep your body needs.

Action Step

Develop a good sleep routine and protect it. Turn off your electronic devices two hours before bedtime.

Closing

We hope you've learned something through our eBook as we have a passion for helping those who desire to live forever young. If you would like more information, please visit our website at www.ForeverYoung.MD.

If you've enjoyed our eBook, please leave feedback. It's only through your insights and support that we will have any success getting our passionate message out to many others. Our sincere contributions to health mean nothing without your support.

Thank you for reading. Keep thriving to the end!

Other Books You May Enjoy

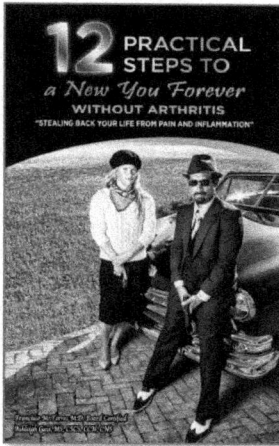

12 Practical Steps to a New You Forever Without Arthritis – *Stealing Back Your Life from Pain and Inflammation*

by Dr. Franscisco M. Torres & Ashleigh Gass

One Size Does NOT Fit All Diet Plan – *Meal Planning That Will Boost Your Metabolism, Break Through Plateaus, and Help You Achieve Maximum Fat Loss Today!*

by Abby Campbell

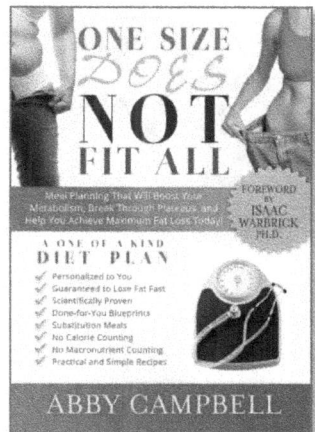

"There is no challenge too large to overcome."

~Dr. Torres